LOVE AND THE DIGNITY OF HUMAN LIFE

Love and the Dignity of Human Life

On Nature and Natural Law

•   •

Robert Spaemann

Foreword by
David L. Schindler

•   •

HUMANUM

WILLIAM B. EERDMANS PUBLISHING COMPANY

GRAND RAPIDS, MICHIGAN / CAMBRIDGE, U.K.

Published 2012 by

Wm. B. Eerdmans Publishing Co.

2140 Oak Industrial Drive N.E., Grand Rapids, Michigan 49505 /

P.O. Box 163, Cambridge CB3 9PU U.K.

www.eerdmans.com

Printed in the United States of America

18 17 16 15 14 13 12   7 6 5 4 3 2

Library of Congress Cataloging-in-Publication Data

Spaemann, Robert.

Love and the dignity of human life: on nature and natural law /
Robert Spaemann; foreword by David L. Schindler.

p.   cm.

"A John Paul II Institute book."

ISBN 978-0-8028-6693-6 (pbk.: alk. paper)

1. Love — Religious aspects — Catholic Church. 2. Dignity —
Religious aspects — Catholic Church. 3. Brain death — Religious
aspects — Catholic Church. 4. Catholic Church — Doctrines.   I. Title.

BV4639.S655   2012

241'.697 — dc23

2011026646

Humanum is an imprint of the
John Paul II Institute for Studies on Marriage and Family
at the Catholic University of America in Washington, D.C.

Contents

Foreword

David L. Schindler

The three essays making up this book were presented as the 2010 McGivney Lectures of the Pontifical John Paul II Institute for Studies on Marriage and Family at The Catholic University of America. The Institute is sponsored by the Knights of Columbus, a Catholic fraternal society founded by Father Michael J. McGivney in 1882 for the purpose of "protecting widows and children of working men and fostering their faith and social progress." In honor of Father McGivney, the Institute periodically invites distinguished Catholic scholars to lecture in the fields of theology, philosophy, and allied disciplines. The lectures, inaugurated with the founding in 1987 of the American

---

David L. Schindler is Provost and Gagnon Professor of Fundamental Theology of the Pontifical John Paul II Institute for Studies on Marriage and Family at The Catholic University of America.

campus of the Lateran University-based Institute, have as their focus any theme bearing significantly on the foundations of human dignity and life: person, family, and community. Previous lecturers have included John Finnis; Elizabeth Anscombe; Ralph McInerny; Kenneth Schmitz; Benedict Ashley, O.P.; Jérôme Lejeune; Cardinal Christoph Schönborn; Cardinal Marc Ouellet; Luis Alonso Schökel, S.J.; Rev. Francis Martin; and Marko Rupnik, S.J.

Robert Spaemann, author of the 2010 lectures, is Professor *Emeritus* of Philosophy at the University of Munich. After studying philosophy, theology, and French literature at Muenster, Munich, and Fribourg, he completed his doctorate in philosophy at the University of Muenster in 1952, under the direction of Joachim Ritter. In 1969 he was appointed professor at the University of Heidelberg (1969-73), where he succeeded Hans Georg Gadamer. In 1973 he joined the distinguished Faculty of Philosophy of the University of Munich, where he remained until his retirement in 1992. He is honorary professor at the University of Salzburg and at the Academy of Social Sciences of China in Beijing, and has been a visiting professor at the Sorbonne, among other universities. Professor Spaemann is the 2001 recipient of the Karl Jaspers Prize of the City and University of Heidelberg and an officer of the Order of the Academic Palms of France; and in 1995 was awarded an honorary doctorate by The Catholic Univer-

David L. Schindler

sity of America, "in recognition of his contribution to philosophy and theology, particularly for his studies of religion and culture." He is at the present time also a member of the Pontifical Academy for Life. Among Professor Spaemann's major works appearing in English are *Basic Moral Concepts* (1989); *Happiness and Benevolence* (2000); and *Persons: The Difference between "Someone" and "Something"* (2007). A translation of his *Philosophische Essays* is soon to be published by ISI Press.

Standing within the great philosophical tradition of the West, Professor Spaemann assists us in thinking through with patience and depth the great questions facing human civilization today. He returns anew to the fundamental questions: Who is a person? What does it mean to speak of personal identity and of the dignity of the person? As Professor Holger Zaborowski notes in his recently published book *Robert Spaemann's Philosophy of the Human Person: Nature, Freedom, and the Critique of Modernity* (Oxford University Press), the first book-length study of Spaemann in English, Spaemann subjects modernity to an interesting and challenging critique, while making clear that we must beware of slipping into a modern anti-modernism which would itself only perpetuate some of the main problematic features of modernity.

In these fascinating essays, Professor Spaemann first treats the "Paradoxes of Love," in which, *inter alia*, he ponders why "'knowing' can only be fulfilled in love": *ubi amor, ibi oculus* ("where love is, there is the eye": Richard of St. Victor); why "to love someone means to understand the reason that God had to create this person" (Nicolás Gómes Dávila); and why "personhood exists only in the plural."

In "Human Dignity and Human Nature," the professor argues that we should not say

> that it is a right to have one's own dignity. Dignity is rather the transcendental ground for the fact that human beings have rights and duties. They have rights because they have duties, i.e., because the normal, adult members of the human family are neither animals who are instinctively integrated into their communities, nor merely instinctually indeterminate subjects of drives. . . . The capacity to assume responsibility is what we call freedom. Someone who is not free cannot be made responsible for anything. But someone who can assume responsibility has the right not to be treated as a mere object or to be physically forced to fulfill his duty.

Further, he says "the preciousness of man 'as such' — that is, 'precious' not only to himself — renders his life something holy, giving the concept of dignity an ontological dimension which is in fact its *sine qua non*. Dignity signals something sacred. The concept is a fundamentally religious-metaphysical one."

In the final essay, Professor Spaemann takes up the difficult issue of whether brain death is the defining criterion for death. The 1968 Harvard Medical School Commission fundamentally changed the *status quaestionis* in this matter when it declared that the death of the brain is indeed the death of the human being. In his essay, Spaemann challenges this conclusion, arguing on the basis of an empirically informed philosophical judgment that "the 'brain death' criterion is only suited to prove the irreversibility of the process of dying and to thus set an end to the physician's duty of treatment as an attempt to delay death," citing German jurist Prof. Dr. Ralph Weber. The brain dead patient, in the words of another German jurist, Prof. Dr. Wolfram Höfing, "is a dying human being, still living in the sense of the Basic Constitutional Law [of the Federal Republic of Germany, ESSJ Art 2, II, I 99]. . . . Brain dead patients have to be correctly regarded as dying, hence living people in the state of irreversible brain failure."

A reviewer of one of Professor's Spaemann's books once said that, if Socrates had written a book, it would have been the book by Robert Spaemann that he was reviewing. What the reviewer meant to convey by these words is manifest in the essays that follow.

The Paradoxes of Love

"We never advance one step beyond ourselves." With this statement, David Hume expressed the heart of the modern worldview. This might become even clearer, if we add the statement of Thomas Hobbes, which says that knowing a thing means "to know what we can do with it when we have it." Consider that the Hebrew *jadah* — the term for "knowing" in the Bible — appears for the first time where it says, "Adam knew his wife and she gave birth to her first son." Aristotle's statement, *intelligere in actu et intellectum in actu sunt idem,* also lives from this insight.[1] Knowing is to become one with the known, while in this unity the known comes into its own. The Cartesian perspective is different. Descartes' prototype of knowledge is the windowless brightness of subjects that stay within themselves,

1. "Knowing in act and the known in act are the same."

which secures their controlling power. Hume's statement expresses that the subject remains in itself and that every notion of self-transcendence or being-outside-of-oneself is an illusion. It is not presently my task to show the logical inconsistency of this statement (if it were true, then it would be impossible to know and express what it says). I would only like to point out that this statement character-izes the mainstream of modern consciousness. This does not mean that all people think this way. Common sense *cannot* think this way. But common sense is unable to find itself anymore in what the official interpreters of reality want us to believe. They want us to believe that we are not what we think we are. They want us to believe that what we understand truth to be does not exist, and likewise for what we mean by the word "love."

But, indeed, does this word mean anything unequivo-cal? Is love a *clara et distincta perceptio*?[2] In fact, there is no word — except maybe "freedom" — that has such a wide-ranging and often contradictory conglomerate of meanings as the word "love." It denotes feelings that par-ents have for their children, and children for their par-ents, and friends for their friends. But especially and above all that famous and never highly enough praised feeling that unites man and woman, and which is used in

2. "Clear and distinct perception."

the Sacred Scriptures of Jews and Christians as a metaphor for the relationship between God and his people, or between God and the one devoted to him. We also speak about love for one's country. When one of Germany's former federal presidents was asked about his love for his fatherland, he answered: "I love my wife, not the state." But this is to distort the question: nobody needs to love the state, in order to love his home-country and fatherland, even to the point of sacrificing his life for it. We also use the term "love" to signify pure sexual desire and its satisfaction. Here, the ambiguity of the term becomes most obvious: the same act of sexual union can be experienced as the deepest expression of love, and as a pure instrumentalization in the service of the crudest egoism. Or, more subtly: the most enthusiastic feeling of love can be a mere means of increasing the intensity of one's own life-experience, the other becoming a mere means of experiencing these feelings, and loved only as long as this drug works. And if, then, the promise of fidelity is broken, absolution comes from the intensity of a new love. As the old tune goes: "How could love be sin?"

At this point, however, I have to question the initially assumed characterization of love as *a feeling.*

On the one hand, this is what it seems to be: if a wife were to ask her husband — or *vice versa* — if he still loved her, and he answered that he loves her, but does not have any feelings for her anymore, then the wife — or the husband — would rightly find this strange. Nevertheless, nobody would say that he did not love his wife this morning, because he did not have the time to think of her all morning long. The lover is a lover insofar as, if he thinks of the beloved person, he thinks of her with love. As a consequence, he loves to think of her, and consequently thinks of her often, and loves to be in her presence. This is precisely what Aristotle calls a *hexis,* and the Latinists a *habitus.*

In this sense, for example, knowledge is a "habit." One does not always have to think of what one knows. But if one thinks of it, one thinks of it with that kind of conviction which we call knowledge. Yet, in the case of knowledge, there is an additional feature that cannot be described at all as merely a mental state, i.e., the conviction that we know, since this conviction can be an error. We only talk of knowledge when things are in fact as we think they are. This is different in the case of love. Yes, I can be deceived in this case, too, but this deception is not a deception about facts in the world, but only a deception about myself.

There is another way in which the habit of love is different from that of knowledge. I know something, if I can situate what I know among all the other things that I know, through reasons. I know it, that is, if I can connect it with the totality of my convictions in such a way that it has become part of my identity. Even then, however, it can be an error. The relation which makes a conviction into knowledge, i.e., the relation of truth, is a purely objective one, which does not touch on or modify at all the mental state of believing that I know. Here, therefore, Hume's statement is indeed in some sense true: "We never advance one step beyond ourselves." Yet, we do want to take this step. The mental state of believing that we know is the belief that we do in fact take this step. Descartes has shown that we can always question this belief again, except for one case where we can be certain that we truly have taken this step, namely when we think or express Hume's statement. We do claim reality for "ourselves," when we deny that step beyond ourselves. "I think" implies "there is thinking," "thinking is happening": not only do I think that I am thinking, but my thinking happens within a space that is larger and wider than the space of my consciousness, and in which my thinking itself occurs as an objective fact. It is the idea of God that opens up this space. Likewise it is the idea of God which allows me to believe that my thinking stands in something like the relation of truth. There is no direct path here to the other of myself, not something like a real contact. Nor does it exist for a Leibnizian monad, dreaming to be with the other; in this case, we are all only life-long dreams, coordinated by God.

This is different in love. What the term "knowing" means can only be fulfilled in love. *Ubi amor, ibi oculus,* we read in Richard of St. Victor.[3] Whether a particular intentional state is a case of knowledge cannot be decided through observation of this state itself, but only through circumstances that are entirely extrinsic to this state. Whether something is a case of love, on the other hand, is decided only from the character of a particular state of mind.

Yet does this not mean that love cannot be placed on the same level as understanding and knowing, i.e., with mental states that transcend themselves, and of whose definition such transcendence is part? *Amor oculus est,* it says in Richard of St. Victor.[4] But popular wisdom has it in the reverse: "love makes blind." Someone in love makes up an image of the beloved that cannot stand the later tests of experience. On the other hand, truly personal love transcends all images, all qualities of the beloved and aims at the person beyond all these qualities. The qualities are that through which love is enkindled. But once it is enkindled it leaves these qualities behind. The one who can answer the question why he loves this person does not yet love truly. The lover is therefore ready and open to

---

3. "Where love is, there is the eye."
4. "Love is an eye."

engage all the future changes of the beloved person, and to tie irrevocably, for better or for worse, his own changes, his own biography, to that of the other. Here we find one of the paradoxes about which I want to talk. The unconditionality of the commitment, the promise of fidelity, is constitutive of love. Here we find another paradox: the case that this promise is not kept happens frequently, very frequently. It is not kept, because the other has changed more than the lover can stand, or because the lover has lost his love "like a stick or a hat." Because the unconditionality and the perspective of unchangeability is constitutive, it appears to the former lover in hindsight as if he had in fact never truly loved — especially if a new love takes away the luster of the old one. Indeed, it is part of the Catholic teaching on love of God and neighbor that no one can never know for sure whether he has it or not.

Of course, one can always know for sure whether one is "in love" or not. This article of the *Catechism* does not speak of infatuation, but of the *habitus* of the *amor benevolentiae*. Now, it is here that we come to the heart of all the paradoxes that occur in the context of the notion of love. It seems that the term does in fact denote two entirely different things, two attitudes, which already Aristotle had distinguished when he speaks of the three types of friendship: that for the sake of pleasure, that for the sake of its usefulness, and that because the friend is worthy of being loved for his own sake.

Tradition then spoke of *amor concupiscentiae* and *amor benevolentiae*.[5] The New Testament calls friendship for the sake of the friend *agape, caritas*. For the one who has friendship with God, every human being is potentially a friend. Yet even here again a paradox creeps in: if every man is a friend, then we need a new term to signify the phenomenon of exclusive friendship, which does not get lost in Christianity, and which, in the Bible, even gives the model for the special relationship between God and the people of God.

On the other hand, *amor concupiscentiae* and *amor benevolentiae* seem to denote such opposite phenomena that we could wonder why the term "love" is used for both of them. The one must have something to do with the other. That they have something to do with each other seems also to be the most important message of the pope's encyclical *Deus Caritas Est,* in which the *amor concupiscentiae* is raised in status by being attributed to God himself: God appears in the prophets as the jealous lover of his bride, the people Israel. In the Incarnation, God even enters the situation of someone who is in need of and dependent on the love of others.

Nevertheless, tradition has avoided the inner oppositions within the concept of love by simply distinguishing two kinds of love, without inquiring about their

5. "Love of concupiscence" and "love of benevolence."

inner unity. Friedrich von Spee in his *Güldenes Tugendbuch*[6] — highly valued by Leibniz — distinguishes between *begierliche Liebe* and *Liebe der Gutwilligkeit*,[7] the latter which he also calls love of friendship. In regard to God he identifies the *amor concupiscentiae* with the virtue of hope, similar to Fénelon, who later will write: "En perdant l'espérance on retrouve la paix."[8] For Spee one can talk about love in the full sense only if both come together. He writes:

> As an example that often both come together, take this: a bridegroom loves his bride with both of these loves, for he loves her with the love of desire, since he desires her for himself and embraces her heartily, who is pleasing to him and, as he thinks, his salvation and delight. He also loves her with the love of benevolence or friendship, since he also wishes her well from his heart, and wants and desires every good for her. On the other hand, one often loves something only with the love of desire and not with the love of benevolence and friendship. Take this example: an evil man might love a woman only with the love of desire, because he

6. *Golden Book of Virtues.*
7. "Desirous love" and "love of benevolence."
8. "Losing hope, one retrieves peace."

only embraces her for his lust and her beauty, while he does not otherwise want for her or wish her any good, but would rather "send her to Jericho," if only he can satisfy his desires. Thus he loves her only with the love of desire and not with the love of benevolence or friendship. In like manner, I, too, love good food, apples or roses with a love of desire alone, but not with the love of benevolence or friendship.

In a different passage, Spee introduces the notion of "pure love," i.e., pure friendship without desire. For this, he chooses examples from the realm of politics — similar again to Thomas Aquinas and later Fénelon: Thomas talks about love of one's fatherland; Fénelon, characteristically, about the love of the citizens for the ancient republics; Spee about the love for the emperor, "our gracious Lord Ferdinand II, whom I do not precisely love with a love of desire, but whom I do love with a strong love of benevolence." This love is then illustrated as an example of selfless love, since the subject does not gain an immediate advantage from the good fortune of the emperor, his victories, etc. He cannot even delight in the sight of his triumph, because the emperor is far away.

But the political examples show that the *amor benevolentiae* without any desire likewise does not exemplify the perfect love that extends from person to person.

There must be an inner, a constitutive, unity between *amor concupiseentiae* and *amor benevolentiae. Philia, amor amicitiae,*[9] is something different from the merely accidental addition of the two elements in our state of mind. Rather, one would have to speak of a dialectic of love. Leibniz has suggested a definition of love, which he later also thought apt to settle the famous *amour pur* debate between Bossuet and Fénelon, a "formula of concord" *(Konkordienformel),* so to speak. His definition is: *delectatio in felicitate alterius.*[10] In this definition, both are contained: first, that love is a state of mind of the lovers, a *delectatio.* This was in contradiction to Fénelon's critique of Jansenism. The Jansenists had spoken of a *delectation supérieure.*[11] They had appropriated Vergil's *trahit sua quamque voluptas.*[12] Whether someone is a child of grace becomes apparent from what he delights in. For Fénelon, on the other hand, the *désintéressement*[13] of love proves itself in the firm adherence of the will, even when the soul in its contact with divine things senses nothing, i.e., when the soul is in the state of dryness which, for the pupils of St. Augustine, was a sign of being

9. Love of friendship.
10. "Delight in the happiness of the other."
11. A higher delight.
12. "Each pleasure draws its own."
13. Disinterestedness.

lost. Love has to do with delight, Leibniz insists on this. But the content of this delight is the happiness of the other. (It is notable, by the way, that Leibniz chooses as his example for this kind of love the delight that we have in viewing a painting of Raphael, even if we neither own this painting, nor want to get any other advantage from it. "Disinterested delight" will be Kant's definition, following Leibniz's definition of aesthetical feelings. The objection, that the example is not well chosen because paintings cannot be happy, is rejected by Leibniz with reference to the fact that *delectatio* is only a subjective form of experience belonging to an objective perfection; hence, one can define love also as the *delectatio in perfectione alterius.*[14] This love, then, can also have a painting of Raphael as its object. This, by the way, does not seem to be a satisfying answer. For personal love aims at something beyond all perceivable qualities, while the delight in the painting only terminates at the qualities, and therefore also does not include any promise of faithfulness, through all the possible changes of the painting.)

Delectatio in felicitate alterius. The definition is not: *delectatio per felicitatem alterius.*[15] This is crucial. If the goal is one's own joy, and the happiness of the other only

14. Delight in the *perfection* of the other.
15. Delight *because of* the happiness of the other.

the means to obtain this joy, then we cannot speak of love. *Delectatio in felicitate alterius* — that means: the delight is not a mere state of the subject, but it has an intentional content, by which it is qualified. It is worthwhile to read, in this context, a little text of the great Arnauld, the *Dissertation sur le prétendu bonheur des plaisirs des sens.*[16] In this text from the middle of the 17th century, Arnauld insists on the intentional character of joy. Joy has not only efficient causes, which, after all, could also be psycho-pharmaceutical causes. Joy has a content, through which it is specifically qualified. The joy about the blooming apple trees in May, the joy about the reunion with a beloved person, the joy about a particular piece of music, do not only have different causes, but they are different joys. Arnauld calls the content of the *delectatio* the *causa formalis,*[17] in contradistinction to the *causa efficiens.*[18] When Thomas Aquinas distinguishes between *beatitudo formalis* and *beatitudo objectiva,* he is concerned about the same issue.[19] The love of God does not love God because he causes in us a state of mental well-being, but he is rather the objective content of this happiness. Hence, the love of God is not about instrumentalizing God as a

16. "Dissertation on the alleged happiness of sense pleasure."
17. Formal cause.
18. Efficient cause.
19. "Formal happiness" and "objective happiness."

means for a goal extrinsic to him, but is about God himself. However, in this self-transcendence we find, at the same time, the fulfillment of our own nature. Fénelon saw in Bossuet such an instrumentalization of God for a basically finite happiness. He himself, on the other hand, described pure love as a passing away, a death of finite nature — whereas Thomas had written that *by nature* each being loves God more than itself, just as every part loves the whole more than itself. Again, it is the love of one's fatherland that serves as the paradigm.

In the 17th century, however, ontology and psychology had drifted so far apart that there was no bridge leading from one to the other. The acceptance of one's own damnation, if it be God's will, is ontologically irrelevant, but it is a stage on the way to the purification of the heart of any egoistic reflection. Indeed, reflection cannot find innocence, but can only unmask every impulse for disinterested activity as a case of subtle self-love. This was also Luther's problem. It is, moreover, obvious in sexual relations. The pleasure of the other is an essential part of one's own pleasure. *Delectatio in felicitate alterius.* Is the interest in the pleasure of the other therefore egoistic? Should the lady whom I honor with a bouquet of flowers accept with the remark: "How nice that you have provided yourself with the pleasure of presenting me such a beautiful bouquet"? We would probably be somewhat frustrated by this reaction. We could, of course, get even with the response: "Well, you know, I actually don't really care whether this makes you happy or not. But I do find it simply correct, i.e., morally good, to give another person pleasure, although I don't have any feelings at all about it." That would undermine the pleasure of gift-giving and gift-receiving. Already La Rochefoucauld had noticed that reflection always finds only self-love — *amour propre* — and not love; but Fénelon finds the reason for it: reflection itself has its motivation in self-love. It is reflection which destroys innocence and can, therefore, only find self-love in searching its own interior. "He who looks at a woman in order to desire her, has already committed adultery with her," says the Gospel. It does not say: "he who looks at a woman *and* desires her," but "he who looks at her, *in order to* desire her." It is the "in order to" by which the one looked at is not herself anymore the object of *amor concupiscentiae,* but rather the desire itself is the goal and the desired person only the means to experience the desire. That is adultery, even if it is one's own wife.

Innocence has something to do with immediacy. Heinrich von Kleist, in his essay on the puppet show, shows how an imperceptible step of reflection destroys the innocence of immediacy. It can only be restored, writes Kleist, if "consciousness has gone through an infinity." Immediacy cannot be regained through an immediate attempt. On the contrary, when immediacy and spontaneity are appealed to, in order to excuse the violation of fidelity and the breaking of a promise — "How could love be sin?" — then immediacy has already been lost. *Corruptio optimi pessima.*[20] Man is the being of reflection, who has always already lost his initial innocence, and he cannot regain it through claiming that spontaneity which is lost precisely by the act of claiming it. It is regained rather in the forsaking of all of these tricks, and in the simple response: "No. Love is never sin. But the violation of a human person is, the violation of fidelity is, and the breaking of a promise is." The phrase, "That is just how I am, and you have to accept me just as I am," is an impertinence, even if it justifies itself theologically with the unspeakable nonsense that God accepts us as we are. If that were true, then there would be no such thing as forgiveness. To say to someone who has done me wrong, "Well, that's just how you are," is the opposite of forgiveness. Forgiveness means not to pin someone down on being what he is — a coward, a liar, or a traitor — but to allow him to distance himself from his being that way, and to begin anew. Being able to do so is characteristic of a person. Because love aims at the person, it can let go of the "that is just how you are," and allow the other to dis-

---

20. "The corruption of the best is the worst."

tance himself from himself and have a new beginning. To accept someone as he is, is the ultimate form of resignation. The proclamation of Jesus does not begin with the words: "God accepts you as you are," but with the words: "Repent, change! Be different from what you are now!"

Love gives the beloved the possibility to be a person, and to be a person in a unique, non-interchangeable way. It is the eyes of the lover that perceive the uniqueness of the beloved, a uniqueness that is more than the combination of empirical qualities. Nicolás Gómes Dávila writes: "To love someone means to understand the reason that God had to create this person." It is in this sense that love gives sight. *Ubi amor, ibi oculus.* Love lets the beloved appear in a glow that nobody else perceives. When this glow slowly fades into the ordinariness of everyday life, then this does not mean that now, slowly, reality appears as it is, but rather the opposite. The lover will retain the memory of the once-perceived glow as the apostles retained the memory of the transfiguration of Christ; and he will know that then true reality was shown to him, the "thing in itself," which, as Kant says, is the thing as it appears to an *intellectus archetypus.* The loving educator, too, needs this gaze, which teaches him to understand the reason why a young person who is entrusted to him exists.

But while I am talking, I am passing over another paradox, or another ambivalence, in the concept of love. The so-called commandment of love in the Gospel refers to all human beings. Each human being is an *imago Dei,* and the one who offers his life for him never does something meaningless in doing so. Mother Teresa did not choose the people for whom she was there; she simply was there for them. Yet, there is an *ordo amoris.*[21] There is a creaturely relation of nearness and distance that is not invalidated by the commandment to love one's neighbor. Peter Singer thinks that, if two children are drowning and I can only save one, then the fact that one of them is my own should not matter for the question as to which one I should save. I would have to save the one who, because of his great talents and special qualities, promises to increase the improvement of the world in a higher degree. This is the attempt to take God's viewpoint and to devalue creaturely relations. As if we know by what the world is improved! It certainly is not improved by people who imagine themselves to bear the responsibility for the universe.

To the contrary, love is by its nature distributed unevenly. There are relations of friendship, which are by their nature exclusive. When St. Benedict in his rule forbade private friendships between monks, he did so because he considered this community of monks as already

21. An order of love.

being a community of friends. The renunciation necessitated by an exclusive relationship of two people has to be
seen in line with the renunciation necessitated by marriage, which normally, like friendship, is seen as being
part of a good human life. Why?

In order to answer this question, let me make a little
detour. One definition of love we find in a text of Valentin
Tomberg says: "Love is the becoming real of the other for
me." Knowledge always subsumes the other under universal concepts. Something can only be identified if it is
identified as a such-and-such. The individual in itself is
an *ineffabile*, and, as Quine has shown, referring to it always remains indeterminate. It always remains less real
for me than I am to myself. The other's toothache is simply less real for me than my own. Buddhism teaches a
way to become just as unreal to ourselves as the others
are to us. Christianity, on the contrary, teaches — as the
religion of love — that the other is just as real as we are. It
teaches one to rejoice with the rejoicing and to weep with
the weeping. The indeterminacy of the reference disappears if the reference is established by the word "thou."
Though I can be mistaken about the qualities of a person,
the identity of a person is not a qualitative, but a numeri-
cal one. And the one who has been addressed as Thou
can answer the speaker and by that confirm that indeed
he is that Someone who has been addressed.

If we converse with many people, then this is possible only through generalizations, i.e., through concepts. The *ineffabile* of the individual person cannot become real for me in the emphatic sense that I have mentioned before. Not around everyone can be that glow that is around those we love. Most people I will perceive only under certain aspects and concepts. Nobody can do justice to the uniqueness of each human person, except God. "Only for God is everyone irreplaceable," says Dávila. Only for God does the individual not disappear in the great number. To become real as this non-interchangeable unique individual — this is possible for me only in the exclusive forms of friendship and love. Nobody can give without taking. That love that can do justice to the uniqueness of the person can only be defended if exclusivity is defended. This is why jealousy is part of the *amor amicitiae.* Pavel Florensky, in his chief work *The Pillars and Foundations of Truth,* dedicated the last of his twenty-two letters to the defense of jealousy. Total absence of jealousy at a given occasion is an insult of the beloved person, who in this is degraded to one among others. That is why especially the Old Testament speaks frequently of the jealousy of God with regard to his people. Not to have alien gods besides him is the first of the Ten Commandments — an expression of jealousy.

However, the exclusive *amor amicitiae* does not in

fact stand in competition with the commandment to love my neighbor, which regards everyone who through circumstances becomes my neighbor. It rather gives this love of neighbor its depth. For everyone has a claim to be recognized as real, and real as this unique person. What everyone is becomes a real experience for us in one person, in the exclusive relation of friendship. It becomes an experience only for that one who enters into this relationship with one person and unites his destiny, for better or for worse, with that of the other. The *amor amicitiae* leaves behind the opposition between desire and benevolence; both are inseparable for it. He who truly wishes another well with all his heart will let him feel that he, the lover, also needs him, the beloved. He who only wants to be the giver does not give enough. Christianity teaches that the ultimate gift of God is that he makes himself into a receiver with regard to us. He who gives someone to understand that he is ready to be everything for him, but that he is not interested in being loved himself, humiliates the other. The *amor benevolentiae* is love only if it is also *amor concupiscentiae.* And the same is true *vice versa.* Someone who really desires the other can only obtain what he desires if he is willing to give. This is true for sexual desire, which finds its true fulfillment only if the other one finds it as well. But it is true also for any other level of life. Epicurus shows that incomparably well, when he writes that a happy life is impossible without a good friend. But we can have a good friend only if we are good friends ourselves. A really good friend, however, is the one who is willing to give his life for his friends. He who truly wants to be happy and content must therefore be ready to give his life for his friend. The wisdom of the hedonists, then, ultimately leads to a statement of the Gospel — if in fact the hedonist has understood the dialectic of the *amor concupiscentiae.*

I am arriving now at a final paradox of the concept of love, the paradox of human sexuality. It is a *topos* of morality that it is one of the tasks of a human being to integrate his sexuality into personal love, and that this is often difficult to achieve. For it seems that something contradictory is asked from us: the highest expression of personal love is supposed to happen precisely in that which is most impersonal, namely sexual relations. In brothels the animal drive, which leads to sexual relations, is satisfied even with total strangers. It is a submersion in the anonymous stream of life as it perpetuates itself. It is here that man takes off the *persona* in the ancient sense of a social role. That is why he typically hides from the sight of third persons; and often he wants to erect a barrier between this sphere and that of the bourgeois world. What he says, swears, and promises in this sphere, must not be taken seriously. It does not count in the social world. Often men and women who have "been intimate" with each other do not want to be seen together outside. European antiquity was relatively promiscuous; yet at the same time ancient philosophy held this sphere in a certain contempt. The sphere in which one can forget oneself was contrasted with the ideal of a life governed by reason. The idea of a person in the Christian sense, who finds his highest actualization in the self-forgetfulness of love, was not yet born. The perversions of Sadism and Masochism live from this idea, because they find their pleasure in destroying it. They do not throw themselves into the self-forgetful ecstasy of the senses, but rather celebrate the objectification and depersonalization as a means of self-enjoyment for the Ego.

These demonic mysteries are the most extreme contrast to the feast of the triumphal breakdown of the barriers of shame between lovers. This feast of love makes visible the paradox of which I am speaking. In it is revealed in a special way the nature of a person. Personhood is not the same as being governed by reason. Reason together with the nature of animal drives is that human nature in which the person appears. The personal way to *have* a nature is the governance of reason in life. The submersion in the pre-personal stream of life can and should become the symbol of self-transcendence in which persons realize themselves. The temporary relinquishing of the governance of reason — which is called very nicely *Beischlaf*[22] in German — is not depersonalization if it is embedded in that unconditional, irreversible, and exclusive mutual self-giving of two persons, indeed of two persons whose different sexual *physis* is already ordered toward such a union. Personhood exists only in the plural. To be a person means to occupy a place in the universal, trans-temporal community of persons. Embedded in such a personal union, the submersion of the self in the act of intercourse becomes a symbolic realization of personal self-transcendence.

Paradox is the mark of the overcoming of abstraction. Only what is abstract is subject to the logic of identities. That is why God in Christianity is not understood as a person, but as a community of persons. Only in this way does the statement "God is love" have an intelligible meaning. In the concrete unity of love, the lovers do not disappear, but rather are elevated to the highest level of their possibilities. Likewise, in Christianity love of God is not understood as if it were a dissolution of the person in God, like a drop submerged in the ocean. In this metaphor, God is thought of only as a substance in which everything finite disappears. Of course, we do compare love

22. Sleeping next to, sleeping with.

with death. *Fortis ut mors dilectio,* it says in the Song of Songs.[23] We speak of overcoming oneself, of self-denial and of dying with Christ. Fénelon has defended this way of speaking, while at the same time insisting on a separation of psychology and ontology. What we experience psychologically as self-denial is ontologically a self-realization and rising of the person. The Gospel expresses it in this way: "He who wants to save his soul will lose it, but he who gives it up, will save it." But this self-transcendence includes the readiness for real death. "No one has greater love than the one who lays down his life for his friends." Life lives on the sacrifice of life.

23. "Strong as death is love."

Human Dignity and Human Nature

Dignity is not a property among other empirical data. Nor should we say that it is a human right to have one's own dignity respected. Dignity is rather the transcendental ground for the fact that human beings have rights and duties. They have rights, because they have duties, i.e., because the normal, adult members of the human family are neither animals who are instinctively integrated into their communities, nor merely instinctually indeterminate subjects of drives, who in the interest of their communities need to be kept under social or police control. Human beings can act based on insight, rationally and ethically, and they have the duty to do so. Article 6 of the German Constitution, for example, says: "The care and education of children are the natural right of the parents and are incumbent on them as their first and foremost duty." That parental rights follow from the capacity of the parents to fulfill their parental duty can be seen from the fact that this right ceases to exist in cases of severe neglect of this duty. The capacity to assume responsibility is what we call freedom. Someone who is not free cannot be made responsible for anything. But someone who can assume responsibility has the right not to be treated as a mere object or to be forced physically to fulfill his duty. A slave has no rights, and so neither does he have duties. The state is a community of free people; slaves can be just as little citizens or subjects of a state as domestic animals. If free will is a mere fiction, then the state has its foundation in a fiction, in a mere "as if." It is important that the citizens never come to know about this, but rather sincerely believe in this "as if."

Human dignity has no biological "reason," but having dignity does come with biological membership in the family of free beings — family relations are also personal relations. Father, mother, sister, brother, grandparents, etc. are — in contrast to animal relations — lifelong roles. It is therefore irrelevant whether an individual member of the family does already have, or still has, or has ever had at all those properties that cause us to speak of persons, i.e., those properties which bring dignity phenomenally to appearance.

Our common saying that human dignity ought to be respected rests on a peculiar ambivalence in the thought of the free subject. From this ambivalence follow two different perceptions regarding that which constitutes a violation of this dignity. This dignity is "inviolable" *(unantastbar),* as is said in the German Constitution; and in the standard commentary on the Constitution, it is rightly said that this is to be understood normatively, not descriptively. "Inviolable," after all, could mean that it is *impossible* to violate something, or it could mean that something *should not* be violated. Both meanings have their common root in the fact that human beings are, on the one hand, persons, free subjects, and as such cannot be touched and violated from the outside. The Christian tradition has as its central symbol the image of someone who is apparently completely bereft of his dignity, someone naked and crucified, but at the same time and precisely as such honored with the deepest possible reverence. The scene in Shakespeare is to be understood thus, when old King Lear, cast out by his daughters and in full decline, is approached by the Earl of Kent, who wishes to enter into his service. When Lear objects that he is a mere nothing, Kent answers: "But you have that in your countenance/which I would fain call master."

Here, royal dignity isn't derived from royal power. Royal dignity does sustain a claim to power, but it exists whether or not this claim is realized. At the lower end of the social scale, too, we find the quality of dignity exemplified. There is a special dignity involved in service, a dignity which prevents its bearer from being a mere functionary. It is this, and not just some general "human dignity," that gives the servant a special sense of his own importance vis-à-vis his master. And civilized humanity has always deemed the office of the hangman undignified, while the man being hanged has a prime opportunity to demonstrate dignity at the moment of his execution, thereby becoming an object of respect.

There are patterns of conduct, actions, and situations, which demonstrate this quality in a special way. There are others in which a hint of dignity would immediately evoke a sense of ridiculous affectation. And then there are yet others to which the character of indignity attaches, as a negative quality, abasing the agent. Indignity can only belong to the actions and attitudes of *persons,* that is to say, of free beings to which we ascribe at least *some* degree of dignity (if we are not to feel a certain acute embarrassment on their account). Resentment, hatred, and fanaticism are attitudes integrally opposed to dignity. The deliberate humiliation of a weaker person is just as undignified as cowering before a stronger one. Human dignity is inviolable to the extent that other people cannot take it from you. Only you can forfeit your own dignity. All that other people can do is to affront your dignity by failing to respect it, in which case they do not succeed in stripping you of your dignity. It was not Maximilian Kolbe and Kaplan Popieluszko who lost their dignity; it was their murderers.

What *can* be taken from the other person, however, is the opportunity for dignified self-presentation. When Roman law prohibited the crucifixion of Roman citizens, this was not only because crucifixion was more painful than beheading. It was chiefly because crucifixion puts the victim in a position exposed to the gaze of all, stripped of the possibility of any kind of self-presentation. The executed victim is confronted by others, while, from his perspective, this confrontation lacks the "self-disclosing" character essential for personal communication. Objectively the situation is undignified. So it was with the stocks. The stocks subjected the offender to a situation of objective indignity. Again and again, Christian art has taken up afresh this "adverse object" (Goethe) so as to highlight the dignity of the crucified one even in this situation of objective indignity. The crucified one thus remains for centuries exposed to our gaze, yet now as an object of worship. The cross is the giant leap toward the radical internalizing of the concept of dignity, toward the awareness of something in the phenomenon of dignity at once veiled and unveiled.

So what do the different ways in which dignity appears have in common? Obviously dignity always has something to do with an inner self-possession independent of circumstance. We should not think of this independence as a strategy of compensation for the weak, as in the attitude of the fox, for whom the grapes are too sour, but rather as an expression of strength, the attitude of someone for whom the grapes are not so important and who can be sure to get them whenever he wants. Only a strong animal appears to us as a suitable paragon of dignity, but only in situations where there is no question of greed. And even then, only an animal that doesn't look as if it has been custom-made for the struggle to survive, for example, the crocodile with its enormous mouth or the gigantic insect with its fearful symmetry. Dignity is about mastering one's existence and then displacing that mastery. In their depiction of Christ, the Gospels highlight his powerlessness, presenting it as voluntary renunciation. And in such a way they highlight his dignity. So before his arrest, when Jesus tells the soldiers, "I am he," they immediately fall to the ground.[1] And when he commands Peter to sheathe his sword, Jesus reminds Peter that, if he wished, he could summon twelve legions of angels to His defense.[2]

On the other hand, however, there are acts capable of

1. John 18:5-11.
2. Matt. 26:53.

violating human dignity. But this can only be the case because human beings are not free subjects floating in empty space. Rather, they have a physical and psychical nature, in which they make themselves manifest and in which they can also be violated, independently of their own will. Let me make a few remarks on this topic.

Freedom is a property of the species *Homo sapiens.* But human nature is not solely characterized by the fact that it is a manifestation of freedom. We could imagine rational beings from other planets, which might come to Earth and encounter human beings whose way of behaving they do not understand. Let us imagine that these beings could not experience pain; they themselves would have other signals that would make them aware of diminished health. For them, however, these signals would merely have a character comparable to that of the blinker in a car, i.e., such that they would not of themselves entail the tendency toward relief. These beings could therefore not understand at all why the intentional inducing of such signals, i.e., the intentional infliction of pain, should be something bad. And if such a being did not know sleep, it could not understand what systematic deprivation of sleep would mean. Almost all the contents of our willing are natural contents, which are given through our contingent human nature. And it is only in this contingent human nature that human dignity is violable. This

33

nature is the nature of a species. That is why human beings can understand the tendencies of other human beings, and why they can evaluate conflicting interests and
bring them to a just adjudication. Otherwise, only the intensity of the wish would count, as eccentric and absurd
as this wish might appear to us. And someone could feel
violated in his human dignity, if the intensity of his wish
were not taken into account. We can evaluate desires and
interests only because we share the same nature. Even
the advocates of euthanasia cannot do without such eval-
uations. If only the suicidal wish were to count, then one
would not be permitted to refuse the wish of a young person, unhappily in love, for active assistance in her suicide. The objection that in such cases it is to be expected
that the person after a while will change her mind can be
rejected by her with the counter-argument: "I do not
want time to erode my identification with this love; I
want to die as the person that I am right now." If it is allowed at all to kill someone at his request, and if the dignity of man consists only in his freedom as completely ab-
stracted from his nature, then it is an impermissible
paternalism to evaluate suicidal wishes of this kind at all.
Why should someone not have the right to die as the one
that he is right now?

I want to remind you of yet another example, this
time a real one: the "cannibal of Rothenburg," who had

the wish to kill someone and eat him afterward and who indeed found someone on the internet who had the complementary wish to be killed and eaten. The whole thing happened. The man was accused of murder. His defense was very simple: *Volenti non fit iniuria.*[3] Nothing happened to anyone that was unwanted by him. The state does not have the right to evaluate such wishes and to punish their fulfillment. If he was punished nevertheless, then it was because the court did indeed evaluate these wishes — and this on the basis of a human nature in which human dignity can be violated, in spite of agreement. If we disapprove of the behavior of the cannibal, then we assume a normative concept of the natural as the "normal."

We cannot do without a concept of normality in our dealings with living things. In the realm of physics there is no such thing as normality; there is only a strict natural law that does not tolerate exceptions. If a planet deviates from its calculated course, then we do not speak of the wrong behavior of the planet, but we feel that we need to correct the parameters of our calculation. In the realm of non-living beings, there is no such thing as right or wrong. But if a rabbit is born with three legs, if a lioness does not teach her young how to hunt their prey, or if for

3. "To one who is willing, no harm is done."

a primate the individuals of the opposite sex do not have that attraction on which the continued existence of the species depends, then we speak of deviations, abnormalities, or defects. The adjustment of animal behavior to its environment presupposes that the animal expects certain behaviors from the other animals, i.e., normality. Likewise we ourselves can find our way in traffic only because we expect that normally other participants in traffic behave normally. And for the same reason we cannot, out of respect for human dignity, treat human beings equally, without regard to their sexual orientation. Someone who hires a pedophile for work in a kindergarten is guilty of negligence. The sexual desire of a pedophile cannot be put on the same level as someone who has a normal sexual orientation. To respect his human dignity does not mean to respect his particular inclinations as an expression of this dignity. Rather, we have to ask of him to forgo definitively the satisfaction of these desires. For their fulfillment would mean an irreparable damage to the psyche of the child, which in turn will prevent it in the future from leading a life that we call "normal." Without this concept of normality we would be unable to answer the question why the interests of the child should have priority over the interests of the pedophile. After all, he, too, could claim to experience damage, if he has to forgo the fulfillment of his desires. The answer cannot be that the interests of a child have priority before those of adults in principle, but rather that both interests are not on the same level. One, the interest in a normal life, is a normal interest, whereas the interest of the pedophile is not.

The still-canonical interpretation of the German Constitution understands respect for human dignity to mean, following Kant, that human beings, in all acts that concern them directly or indirectly, are never to be treated merely as means, but always also as ends. It is important to note the "merely." For human beings can live in societies only by continuously treating each other as means to ends. A violation of human dignity occurs only when someone is reduced to this function in other people's interest, and if the mutuality of this kind of instrumentalization is excluded. This is the case, for example, in so-called "unethical contracts" *(sittenwidrige Vertrage)*. Someone can, by virtue of his freedom, dispose of himself. I can make promises that dispose of the rest of my life, for example, in marital or religious vows. But in our legal order such contracts have to be revocable as a matter of civil law. This is why, for example, a contract of unilateral subjection, by which someone is surrendering himself to slavery and, definitively and with intended legal force, renouncing his right to change his mind, is null and void. Here, the state is protecting freedom against the very man himself, who is ready to renounce it. This renunciation is possible. It can even be the highest expression of freedom. The Church can treat these promises as irreversible and so insist on the freedom of man by which he is able to dispose of his whole life. It is important, on the one hand, that the Church cannot use the arm of the state to enforce this human right. On the other hand, the state's protection of marriage is not only concerned with individuals, but also with the institution itself, which is constituted through the consent of a man and a woman and is of great importance to their offspring. The state should not prosecute marital infidelity; but neither does it have to give legal approval to divorce and thus invent the right of a man to give his name successively to several living women. In other words, the state does not need to call, and should not call, concubinage marriage.

The human person has a temporal dimension beginning and ending at some point in time. It is one of the peculiar marks of human persons to have a biography; they can, across long spans of time, identify with any stage of their natural existence. We say, for example, "I was begotten at this time," "my parents thought about aborting me," "I was born at that time," "I possibly will not be clearly conscious in old age," or "I was unconscious at this particular time." The personal pronoun "I" does not refer to "an Ego" — this is an invention of philosophers — but to a natural organism that began to exist as soon as a genetic code originated that was different and independent from the organism of the mother, and that started to unfold continuously and autonomously from the moment of conception. The human person possesses a temporal dimension, a *temporal shape (Zeitgestalt),* and this is respected, insofar as it represents the Absolute, by ensuring that its beginning and end are not the result of intentional making by other human beings. Similarly, to extend life artificially, to reduce the human existence in its final stage to a function of instruments, cheats us of the dignity proper to "dying well" just as much as violent termination. Indeed, violent termination originates from the same spirit as violent extension. It is no different with the beginning of life: our temporal shape is also respected insofar as our beginning is not the work of human hands, but rather occurs by way of a human act which does not take the creation of a product as its primary goal. Only in this way can a human being come to life in his own right, "by nature," as a creature of God, or at least of nature, yet not of his parents. *Genitum non factum:* begotten, not thrown together in a test-tube.

The human person is not an aggregate of the states through which it passes; rather, it is the same identical person that passes through these states. Kant stated this point precisely when he wrote: "Because that which is begotten is a person and because it is impossible to have a concept of the begetting of a free being by means of a physical operation, therefore it is in a practical respect a quite correct and necessary idea to regard the act of conception as one in which we bring a person without his consent into the world and transfer him here by our own will." With regard to the end of life, however, the notion of human dignity is often used in the context of euthanasia and dignified human dying understood to mean suicide. I do not want to discuss here what the correct moral and legal judgment on suicide should be. It is absurd to punish attempted suicide. But it is likewise absurd to speak of a "right to suicide." The truth of the matter is, someone who kills himself withdraws from the web of social relations within which alone we can speak of rights. He steps out of the sphere of law. To be able to do so — not *actually* to do it — is characteristic of what it means to be a person. It is quite different with assisted suicide on demand. This is not an act outside but within the order of right and law; it needs to remain prosecuted by criminal law. Making suicide a right has grievous consequences, for then the bearer of this right is responsible for all the consequences, all the personal and financial burdens, which arise from the fact that he does not make use of this right. From this derives with logical necessity an illegitimate pressure on those who are old or sick. The patient can be free from this responsibility only if he does not have any legal possibility to obtain his death from others at all. No human being can ask from another to declare: "You ought not to exist anymore." An irreversible contract of one-sided submission is an unethical contract and therefore without legal force. A contract for the sake of being killed is completely irreversible as soon as it is executed. It is, therefore, to a much higher degree an "unethical contract" than the one by which someone enters slavery. The term "liberation" is inappropriate for such an act, for the end and goal of any act of liberation is freedom. The end and goal of the act of killing on demand, however, is the elimination of the subject of any possible freedom, his non-existence. But existence is not a property; we don't become poorer by losing it. If we no longer exist, we can no longer suffer loss. Only two things can change this: either a human being survives his own physical death, so that the victim of injustice lives on. Or there exists the God of whom the Psalm speaks, "Precious in the sight of the LORD is the death of his saints."[4] The preciousness of man "as such" — that is, not only precious to himself — renders his life something holy, giving the concept of dignity an ontological dimension which is in fact its *sine qua non.* Dignity signals something sacred. The concept is a

4. Ps. 116:15.

41

fundamentally religious-metaphysical one. Horkheimer and Adorno saw this clearly when they wrote that the only argument against murder is a religious one. This was not, of course, employed as an argument for murder, but rather for taking a religious view on reality. It is a mistake that persists into our own time to think you can drop your religious view on reality without losing something else, something you would not so readily choose to do without.

Dying with true human dignity, on the other hand, is the one who is accompanied by human presence, sheltered and saved from great pain. It is just as much against human dignity to prolong human life beyond any reasonable measure by medical procedures like artificial nutrition against one's own will as it is against human dignity to bring about death intentionally. In either case the patient is no longer truly an "end in itself." This, however, is of crucial importance when it comes to human dignity. Human rights are not absolute: they can limit each other. For example, the right to free research or the right of artistic freedom is limited by property rights. The artist is not allowed to paint on walls that he does not own. A researcher must not seize property in the interest of research, or sacrifice human life. The right to property in turn has its limitations as well. Human dignity, on the other hand, is not subject to compromises. Even when rights are going to be limited, this dignity will insist that, with regard to the considerations of justice that demand or allow these limitations, the question must be asked whether the interests of those whose rights are so limited are impartially taken into account. Human dignity will demand, in other words, that these limitations can be justified as reasonable to those that are negatively impacted by them, provided that those in question are themselves thinking justly. Human dignity can never be in conflict with human dignity. If my interests are to be overridden by those of someone else, then this is no violation of my dignity as long as this infringement can be justified to me.

But a human being is one who can stand back and relativize himself. He can, as Christian terminology has it, "die to himself." Put differently, he can submit his own interests and agendas to a wider conversation because he can recognize other people's interests and agendas as being worthy of equal consideration, while also taking into consideration the position and differences of each. He does not simply make everything a feature of his own environment. On the contrary, he realizes that he himself constitutes an environment for other things and other people. In thus relativizing his own finite "I," his own desires, interests, and intentions, the person expands to become open to the Absolute. He becomes incommensurable and able to offer himself in the service of interests not immediately his own, even up to the point of self-sacrifice. And so the person becomes capable of "love of God carried as far as contempt of self," as Augustine says, a possibility in which he becomes an absolute end-in-himself (not as a natural being but as a potentially moral one). For, since a person can relativize his own interests, he may demand to be respected in his absolute status as subject. Since he himself can freely assume obligations, nobody has the right to make a slave of him, for a slave, as Kant rightly saw, can have no obligations to his master. For one reason and one reason only human beings possess what we call "dignity," because as moral beings they represent the Absolute.

The dignity of a human person is violated in those cases in which it is stated implicitly or explicitly that this person does not count. Thus the Kantian formula of the "end-in-itself" can be restated in a simplified manner: *everyone counts.*

The author is indebted to Guido de Graaff and James Mumford for their translation of "Human Dignity," which appears in *Essays in Anthropology,* published by Wipf and Stock (2010), and which is partly identical to this essay.

Is Brain Death the Death
of a Human Person?

I

Death and life are not primarily objects of science. Our primary access to the phenomenon of life is self-awareness
and the perception of other humans and other living beings. Life is the being of the living *(vivere viventibus est esse),*
says Aristotle. For a living being, not to live means ceasing
to exist. Being, however, is never an object of natural science. It is in fact the *primum notum* of reason and as such
secondarily an object of metaphysical reflection. Because
life is the being of the living, then, life cannot be defined.
According to the classical adage *ens et unum convertuntur,*[1]
it holds true for every living organism that it is alive precisely as long as it possesses internal unity. Unlike the unity

---

1. "Being and unity are convertible."

of atom and molecule, the unity of the living organism is constituted by an anti-entropic process of integration. Death is the end of this integration. With death, the reign of entropy begins — hence, the reign of "destructuring," of decay. Decomposition can be stopped by means of chemical mummification, but this way of preserving a corpse merely holds its parts together in a purely external, spatial sense. Supporting the process of integration with the help of technical appliances, however, is very different. The organism preserved in this way would in fact die on its own if left unsupported, but since it is kept from dying, it is kept alive, and cannot be declared dead at the same time. In this sense Pope Pius XII declared that human life continues even when its vital functions manifest themselves with the help of artificial processes.

II

We cannot define life and death, because we cannot define being and non-being. We can, however, discern life and death by means of their physical signs. Holy Scripture, for example, regards breath as the basic phenomenon of life, and for this reason breath is often simply identified with life itself. The cessation of breathing and heartbeat, the "dimming of the eyes," *rigor mortis,* etc. are the criteria by which, since time immemorial, humans have seen and felt that a fellow human being is dead. In European civilization it has been customary and prescribed by law for a long time to consult the physician at such times, who has to confirm the judgment of family members. This confirmation is not based on a different, scientific definition of death, but on more precise methods to identify the very phenomena already noted by family members. A physician may still be able to discern slight breathing, which escapes a layperson. Besides, the physician could nowadays point out the person whose heart has stopped beating may very well still exist. Due to such sources of error in the perception of death, it is a reasonable traditional rule to let some time elapse between noting these phenomena and the funeral or cremation of the deceased. Similarly, consulting a physician serves the purpose of making sure that a human being is not prematurely declared dead, i.e., non-existent.

III

The 1968 Harvard Medical School declaration[2] fundamentally changed this correlation between medical sci-

---

2. "A Definition of Irreversible Coma. Report of the Ad Hoc Committee of the Harvard Medical School to Examine the Definition of Brain Death," *Journal of the American Medical Association* 205 (1968): 337-340.

ence and normal interpersonal perception. Scrutinizing the existence of the symptoms of death as perceived by common sense, science no longer presupposes the "normal" understanding of life and death. It in fact invalidates normal human perception by declaring human beings dead who are still perceived as living. Something quite similar happened once before, in the 17th century, when Cartesian science denied what anyone can see, namely that animals are able to feel pain. These scientists conducted the most horrible experiments on animals and claimed that expressions of pain, obvious to anyone, were merely mechanical reactions.

This incapacitation of perception fortunately did not last. It is returning today in a different shape, however: namely by the introduction of a new definition of death, or rather the introduction of a definition of death in the first place, in order to be able to declare a human being dead sooner. By the same logic, it would also be possible to define pain in terms of the neurological processes which constitute its "infrastructure," and consequently to define everyone as pain-free for whom these diagnostic findings cannot be confirmed. It is merely a matter of transforming the explanation of pain into a definition, in order to be rid of it as pain. Just like pain, its foundation, life, is equally undefineable. The hypothesis that the total loss of all brain functions immediately and instantaneously brings about the death of a human being frequently eludes discussion in scientific debates by being transformed into a definition: if the death of a human being and the loss of all brain functions are by definition equated, any criticism of this hypothesis is naturally bound to go nowhere. What remains to be asked is whether what is defined in this way is really what all human beings have been used to call "death," as when Thomas Aquinas, in proving the existence of a Prime Mover, a non-contingent Being, etc., concludes his proof with the words: "And this is what all mean when they say 'God.'"

Is "brain death" what all mean when they say "death"? Not according to the Harvard Commission of 1968. The commission intended to provide a new definition of death, one that clearly expressed their main interest. This interest was no longer that of the dying, namely to avoid being declared dead prematurely, but rather that of other people interested in declaring a dying person dead as soon as possible. Two reasons are given in support of this third-party interest: (1) guaranteeing legal immunity for discontinuing life-prolonging measures that would constitute a financial and personal burden for family members and society alike, and (2) collecting vital organs for the purpose of saving the lives of other human beings through transplantation. These two interests are not the patient's interests, since they aim at eliminating him as a subject of his own interests as soon as possible. Corpses are not subjects of interest anymore. The first of the two interests mentioned is incidentally bound to an erroneous premise and a correspondingly problematic practice of the judiciary. It presupposes that for every human being not declared dead, life-prolonging measures are indicated always and without exception. When this premise is dropped, the interest in declaring death at an early point ceases to exist. What remains is the second interest, which is self-contradictory, insofar as it requires on the one hand the collection of live organs, for which reason the dying person needs to be kept alive artificially, while on the other hand it requires that the dying person be declared dead, so that the collection of those organs does not have to be considered an act of killing.

IV

The fact that a certain hypothesis regarding the death of a human being is in the interest of other people who would benefit from the verification of this hypothesis does not prove its falsity. It should cause us, however, to be extremely critical, and it requires setting the burden of proof for this hypothesis very high. This holds true all the more so when the hypothesis is underhandedly immunized by being turned into a definition. Precisely because nominal definitions are neither true nor false, the question of whose interests they serve gains relevance. The strategy of immunization by definition thus has a counterproductive effect.

The legislation of my country allows for a physician's conflict of interests, insofar as, prior to a transplantation, death has to be determined by physicians who themselves are not involved in the transplantation. Unfortunately, however, transplantation physicians did have their share in drafting the Harvard Commission's criteria for the determination of death. It ought to be in the moral interest of transplantation physicians, regarding their own personal integrity, to have as little to do with the formulation of these criteria as with their application, even if this is not in the professional interest of transplantation medicine — although the professional interest of transplantation medicine, considered in itself, is a highly moral interest, the interest of saving the lives of human beings. It has to be ensured, however, that saving lives does not happen at the expense of the lives of other people.

It is a fact that since 1968, the consensus about the new definition of death has not been consolidated; to the contrary, objections against it have increased. Ralf Stoecker states in his 1999 habilitation thesis *Der Hirntod*

("Brain Death") that the switch-over from cardiac death to "brain death" is more contested today than thirty years ago.[3] The arguments against "brain death" are brought forward not only by philosophers, and, especially in my country, by leading jurists, but also by medical scientists, e.g., the American neurologist Alan Shewmon, prominent as a radical advocate of "brain death" still in 1985, until his own medical research convinced him of the opposite.

V

The observer of this discussion is bound to discover that it suffers from a marked asymmetry. The proponents of the new definition argue from a "position of strength." They feel that it is an unreasonable demand to waste more time with arguments, aware that they have the "normative power of the factual" on their side, i.e., an established medical practice which meanwhile has already become routine, as well as, for believers, the blessing of the Church (which, however, was categorically called into question by a public statement of the Cardinal Arch-

3. R. Stoecker, *Der Hirntod. Ein medizinethisches Problem und seine moralphilosophische Transformation* (Freiburg/München: Verlag Karl Alber, 1999), p. 37.

bishop of Cologne). They do not even remotely make the same effort dealing with the arguments of their critics as *vice versa*. Consequently, for every unbiased observer the weight of the arguments has shifted more and more in favor of the skeptics. I myself have to confess that the skeptics' arguments have meanwhile convinced me. Life and death are not the property of science, hence it is the duty of scientists to convince ordinary laypeople of their point of view. When scientists refuse to make this effort under the assumption that they can use arguments from authority instead, their case is indeed in a sorry state. In the following, I would like to make my own argument against the new definition of death. What this definition defines as death is not *quod omnes dicunt mortem*.[4]

VI

The proponents of the thesis that the loss of all brain functions is identical with the death of the human being divide into two separate subgroups. The first group distinguishes between the life of the human being and human life, i.e., the life of a person. According to this group, the term "human life" should only be used as long as

4. "What all mean when they say 'death'."

mental processes of a specifically human nature can be discerned. When the organic basis of such processes ceases to exist, the human being is no longer a person, hence his or her organism is at other persons' disposal to use for their purposes. Consequently, a total loss of all brain functions is not even required at all. Sufficient is the failure of those brain areas that constitute the "hardware" for these mental acts. People in persistent vegetative state are thus considered dead as persons. Not only is this position incompatible with the doctrines of most high religions, in particular Judaism and Christianity, but it also contradicts the tenets of today's medical orthodoxy. A well-known proponent of this position is Australian bioethicist Peter Singer.

The second group starts from the assumption that we can only speak of the death of a human being when the human organism as whole has ceased to exist, i.e., when the integration process constituting the unity of the organism has come to an end. According to this second group, this process of integration is terminated with the total loss of all brain functions, since the brain is assumed to be the organ responsible for integration. Hence, according to the views of this group, the death of the brain is the death of the human being. If the underlying hypothesis is correct, the conclusion must be correct, and even the Church would have no reason to defy this conclusion. But obviously the hypothesis is not correct, and those who wish to adhere to the conclusion are consequently forced to draw closer to the unorthodox theory of the first group, i.e., the cortical death hypothesis.

VII

The hypothesis of at least extensional identity of the total loss of brain functions and the death of the human being is incorrect for several reasons. First of all, it contradicts all appearances, i.e., normal human perception, similar to the Cartesian denial of pain in animals. A German anesthesiologist speaks for many others when she writes that "Brain-dead people are not dead but dying," and that even after thirty years in the profession she could not convince herself of the opposite of what everybody can see. One of the most well-known German neurologists, Prof. Dichgans, head of the Neurologische Universitätsklinik in Tubingen, told me recently that he personally was not prepared to diagnose death based on standard neurological criteria, and therefore did not participate in the determination of death. German intensive care physician Peschke reports that, according to his investigations, nurses in transplantation units are prepared neither to donate their own organs nor to receive donated organs. What they see on a daily basis makes it impossible for them to become part of this practice themselves. One of these nurses writes: "When you stand right there, and an arm comes up and touches your body or reaches around your body — this is terrifying." And the fact that the allegedly dead person is usually given anesthesia, so that the arm stays down, does not contribute to putting less trust in one's own senses. Does one anesthetize corpses? This is merely a suppression of vegetative responses, the argument goes. Yet a body capable of vegetative responses requiring complicated coordination of muscle activity is obviously not in that state of disintegration which would entitle us to say that it is not alive, i.e., that it does not exist anymore.

VIII

Here the reasons of common sense converge with those advanced by medical science. Thus it was already pointed out by Dr. Paul Byrne in 1979 that it is unjustified to equate the irreversible loss of all brain functions with "brain death," i.e., with the end of the existence of the brain.[5] We do not equate the cessation of heartbeat with

5. Paul A. Byrne, Sean O'Reilly, Paul M. Quay, "Brain Death — An Opposing Viewpoint," *Journal of the American Medical Association* 242 (1979): 1985-1990.

the destruction of the heart, because we know today that in some cases this loss of function is reversible. But it is only reversible because the heart precisely does not cease to exist when it ceases to function. And only because the cessation of breathing was not equated with the "death of the lung" did it became possible to utilize mechanical ventilators to restart those functions.

Based on considerations of this kind, Dr. Peter Safar and others began to work on the resuscitation of brain function in brains considered dead by standard criteria. The reply by some that the loss of function in these "resuscitated" brains had not yet become irreversible makes for a circular argument. Irreversibility is obviously not an empirical criterion, since it can always be determined only retrospectively. It is precisely because we assume that the brain still exists that we try to resuscitate its function.

Similarly circular is the reasoning behind the question as to what constitutes "total loss of brain function." The proponents of "brain death" reject the substitution of this term by "loss of all brain functions" on the grounds that this would also pertain to "peripheral brain functions" which can survive the death of the brain as a whole. What are such "peripheral functions"? The Minnesota criteria for this are different from the British criteria, and some authors already declare brain stem activity peripheral when the cortex has ceased functioning. Anything can apparently be regarded as peripheral which is not identical with the integrative function of the brain for the organism as a whole. But the question has precisely been to prove just this integrative functional. So Paul Byrne's words are arguably still valid: "There is no limit to what real functions may be declared peripheral when the only non-peripheral function is imaginary."[6]

IX

Is it justified to call the somatically integrative function of the brain "imaginary"? Among the authors who claim this and give reasons for their views, maybe the most important one is Alan Shewmon. A summary of his empirical research and theoretical considerations can be found in his essay "The Brain and Somatic Integration: Insights into the Standard Biological Rationale for Equating 'Brain Death' with Death."[7] Here I will only present the abstract

6. Paul A. Byrne and Walt F. Weaver, "'Brain Death' Is Not Death," Fourth International Symposium on Coma and Death, Havana, Cuba, March 9-12, 2004.

7. A. Shewmon, "The Brain and Somatic Integration: Insights into the Standard Biological Rationale for Equating 'Brain Death' with Death," *Journal of Medicine and Philosophy* 26 (2001): 457-478.

of this essay, which of course contains neither empirical evidence nor theoretical arguments, only the theses.

> The mainstream rationale for equating "brain death" (BD) with death is that the brain confers integrative unity upon the body, transforming it from a mere collection of organs and tissues to an organism as a whole. In support of this conclusion, the impressive list of the brain's myriad integrative functions is often cited. Upon closer examination and after operational definition of terms, however, one discovers that most integrative functions of the brain are actually not somatically integrating, and, conversely, most integrative functions of the body are not brain mediated. With respect to organism-level vitality, the brain's role is more modulatory than constitutive, enhancing the quality and survival potential of a presupposed living organism. Integrative unity of a complex organism is an inherently nonlocalizable, holistic feature involving the mutual interaction among all the parts, not a top-down coordination imposed by one part upon a passive multiplicity of other parts. Loss of somatic integrative unity is not a physiologically tenable rationale for equating BD with death of the organism as a whole.[8]

8. Ibid., p. 457.

From the actual text of Dr. Shewmon's essay I will only quote a short paragraph:

> Integration does not necessarily require an integrator, as plants and embryos clearly demonstrate. What is of the essence of integrative unity is neither localized nor replaceable — namely the anti-entropic mutual inter-action of all the cells and tissues of the body, mediated in mammals by circulating oxygenated blood. To as-sert this non-encephalic essence of organism life is far from a regression to the simplistic traditional cardio-pulmonary criterion or to an ancient cardiocentric no-tion of vitality. If anything, the idea that the non-brain body is a mere "collection of organs" in a bag of skin seems to entail a throwback to a primitive atomism that should find no place in the dynamical-systems-enlightened biology of the 1990s and twenty-first cen-tury.[9]

X

A nonmedical person, trained in the theory of science and wishing to form an objective opinion about the *status quaestionis,* must strive to evaluate the arguments

9. Ibid., p. 473.

brought forth in the debate. Where results of empirical research are concerned which he or she has no way of verifying independently, it is necessary to confront them with the counter-arguments. Insofar as these counter-arguments are of an empirical nature as well and challenge the accuracy of the presented research results, he or she ought to abstain from judgment until further empirical verification. As far as a theoretical interpretation of the results is concerned, however, he or she is qualified to verify and evaluate it. Regarding the findings presented by Dr. Shewmon, I am not aware of any criticism targeting the core of his argumentation. I conclude from two facts that such criticism indeed does not exist:

(1) When Shewmon presented his research results at the Third International Symposium on Coma and Death in 2000,[10] which was attended largely by neurologists and bioethicists, there was surprisingly broad acceptance. What ensued was a shift of the domain of the debate from the medical to the philosophical arena, with the defenders of "brain death" appealing exclusively to consciousness-based concepts of personhood rather than the previously standard medical rationale of bodily integrity.

10. D. A. Shewmon, "Seeing Is Believing: Videos of Life 13 Years after 'Brain Death,' and Consciousness Despite Congenital Absence of Cortex," Third International Symposium on Coma and Death, Havana, Cuba, February 22-25, 2000.

(2) In 2002, the *National Catholic Bioethics Quarterly* published an article by editor-in-chief Edward J. Furton which was dedicated exclusively to the debate with Alan Shewmon.[11] In this article, Dr. Shewmon's empirical research results are not disputed, nor is any reference made to literature which would justify such doubts. From this I conclude that indeed there is no such literature.

All the more interesting is Furton's argument itself, which defends the equation of "brain death" with death against Shewmon. I will conclude my own remarks with a critical report about this article, beginning with a summary.

Furton's primarily philosophical arguments in favor of "brain death" convinced me more than anything else of the opposite of his position. The reason is that Furton is only able to sustain his thesis of "brain death" as the death of the human being by distinguishing between the death of the human being as a person and the death of the human being as a living being. He writes: "Although the difference between the death of the person and the decay of the body had long been obvious, it is only in our time that the difference between the life of the person and the life of the body has be-

11. E. J. Furton, "Brain Death, the Soul and Organic Life," *National Catholic Bioethics Quarterly* 2, no. 3 (Autumn 2002): 455-470.

come apparent."[12] This, now, is exactly the position of Peter Singer, and it is incompatible with the belief of most religions, and certainly with that of Christianity. If Church authorities cautiously accepted the premise of "brain death," this was always done under the premise that the brain is responsible for somatic integration, the loss of the brain functions thus being identical with the death of the organism. It is beyond the scope of religious authority to judge the validity of this premise. When the premise becomes doubtful, the conclusion ceases to apply.

Furton would like to hold on to the conclusion, even though he abandons the premise under the impression of Alan Shewmon's arguments. His appeal to papal authority is, therefore, unjustified, and it is surprising that he makes such excessive use of the argument from authority in his debate with Shewmon. Just because the Pope bases his own equally hypothetical conclusion on a scientific hypothesis does not mean that this hypothesis is thereby withdrawn from further scientific discourse.

If it were otherwise the Ptolemaic worldview would have been dogmatized forever, just because the Church drew conclusions with religious and practical relevance from it while it was generally accepted. At the same time

12. Ibid., p. 467.

Furton himself concedes in his essay that "the determination of death does not fall under the expertise of the Church, but belongs to the physician who is trained in this field."[13] (I would like to render this more precisely: the physician is qualified to determine the existence of pre-defined criteria for death. The discourse about these criteria themselves falls into the domain of philosophers and philosophizing theologians after they have received the necessary empirical information from the medical profession.) Furton bases his argument on the Aristotelian-Thomistic doctrine of the soul in connection with the teaching of the Church, dogmatized after the Council of Vienne 1311-1312, according to which the human soul is only one, from which follows that the *anima intellectiva* is at the same time the *forma corporis*.[14] From this doctrine, however, Furton draws a conclusion which is diametrically opposed to the intention of St. Thomas as well as the Council of Vienne.

Thomas assumes that the human being initially possesses a vegetative and then an animal soul, and that the spiritual soul is created only on the fortieth day of pregnancy, and not in parallel with the other two souls but in their stead, so that it is now the spiritual soul that simulta-

13. Ibid., p. 463.
14. "Intellectual soul" and "form of the body."

neously fulfills the vegetative and sensorimotor functions. This is drastically different from Aristotle, for whom *nous,* reason, is not part of the human soul, but is *thyrathen,* entering the human being from outside. St. Thomas, by the way, excludes Jesus Christ explicitly from successive animation: that the Incarnation occurs at the moment of his conception presupposes that Jesus' soul must have been a human soul in the full sense from the very beginning. The Church, herein following science, has given up the idea of successive animation long ago and regards not only Jesus, but any human being as a person from the moment of conception, with his or her soul being an *anima intellectiva* — even though the newborn infant is not yet capable of intellectual acts. This inability is due to the lack of sufficiently developed somatic "infrastructure." Similarly, a pianist "cannot" play the piano when there is no piano available. Just as the pianist nonetheless remains a pianist, the soul of the human being is an *anima intellectiva* even when it is factually unable to think. The being of man is not thinking but living: *vivere viventibus est esse.*

Furton's way of thinking is radically nominalistic. For him, a personal soul exists only as long as an individual is capable of specifically personal acts. For Furton, then, the reality of the human soul is not found in allowing man to exist as a living being; the soul is not the *forma corporis* but the form of the brain and only indirectly the form of the body. "The soul is . . . what enlivens a material organ, namely the brain, and from there enlivens the rest of the human body."[15] (This view was rejected already in 1959 by the Würzburg-based neurologist Prof. Joachim Gerlach, for whom the error in the equation of "brain death" and the death of the individual consists in "regarding the brain as the seat of the soul." Similarly, Paul Byrne wrote already in 1979: "'Brain function' is so defined as to take the place of the immaterial principle or soul of man.")[16] Furton identifies that which Thomas calls *intellectus* with factual intellectual consciousness. He does not conclude from the obvious continued existence of a living human organism that the personal soul, which is the form of the human body, is still alive, but contrariwise: if a human being is not capable of intellectual acts anymore, the soul has left him and he is, as a person, dead. The fact that the organism as a whole is obviously still living doesn't play any role. Without actual brain function, the human organism is nothing other than a severed organ, which also still shows expression of life. This position is consequent to, and largely coincides with, that of Peter Singer and Derek Parfit, for whom persons exist only as long as they are capable of personal acts: hence sleeping people, e.g., are not persons.

15. Ibid., p. 470.
16. Cf. Byrne, "Brain Death — An Opposing View Point."

XI

Under the weight of the arguments of Shewmon and others, the group of medically and theologically "orthodox" defenders of "brain death" is apparently disintegrating. In the light of the untenability of the thesis of the integrative function of the brain, the identification of "brain death" and the death of the human being can only be held up if the personality of man is disconnected from being a human in the biological sense, which is what Singer, Parfit, and Furton are doing. To do this under reference to the doctrine of St. Thomas is absurd indeed. Furton avails himself of an equivocation in the term *intellectus* when he claims that being a human consists in the connection of intellect and matter, as though Thomas understood "intellect" in terms of actual thinking rather than the capacity to think. This capacity belongs to the human soul, and this soul is *forma corporis* as long as the disposition of the body's matter permits it. Instead of concluding: where there is no longer any thinking, the *forma corporis* of the human being has disappeared, we can thus only conclude: as long as the body of the human being is not dead, the personal soul is also still present. Only the second conclusion is compatible with Catholic doctrine as well as the tradition of European philosophy. Furton's adventurous conclusion, to declare a human being dead

67

when his or her specifically human attributes do not manifest themselves anymore, is contrary to all immediate perception. Even Peter Singer and Derek Parfit are still closer to the phenomena when they do declare the person expired, but do not already for this reason consider the human being dead.

I conclude with the words of three German jurists who wrote after immersing themselves in the medical literature: "To be correct, the 'brain death' criterion is only suited to prove the irreversibility of the process of dying and to thus set an end to the physician's duty of treatment as an attempt to delay death. In this sense of a treatment limitation, the 'brain death' criterion is nowadays likely to find general agreement" (Prof. Dr. Ralph Weber, Rostock).

"The brain dead patient is a dying human being, still living in the sense of the Basic Constitutional Law [of the Federal Republic of Germany, ESSJ Art 2, II, 1 99]. There is no permissible way to justify under constitutional law why the failure of the brain would end human life in the sense of the Basic Constitutional Law. Accordingly, brain dead patients have to be correctly regarded as dying, hence living people in the state of irreversible brain failure" (Prof. Dr. Wolfram Höfeing, Bonn).

"It is impossible to adhere to the concept of 'brain death' any further. . . . There is no dogmatic return to the days before the challenges to the concept of 'brain death'" (Dr. Stephan Rixen, Berlin).

XII

After all that has been said, for anybody who is still doubtful, the principle applies, according to Hans Jonas, *in dubio pro vita.*[17] Pius XII himself declared that, in case of insoluble doubt, one can resort to presumptions of law and of fact. In general, it will be necessary to presume that life remains.[18]

17. "When in doubt, favor life."

18. Pius XII, *To an International Congress of Anesthesiologists,* Nov. 24, 1957, in *The Pope Speaks* 4, no. 4 (1958): 393-398.